Loving Your Liver

Your Complete Guide to Prevent, Cure and Reverse Fatty Liver

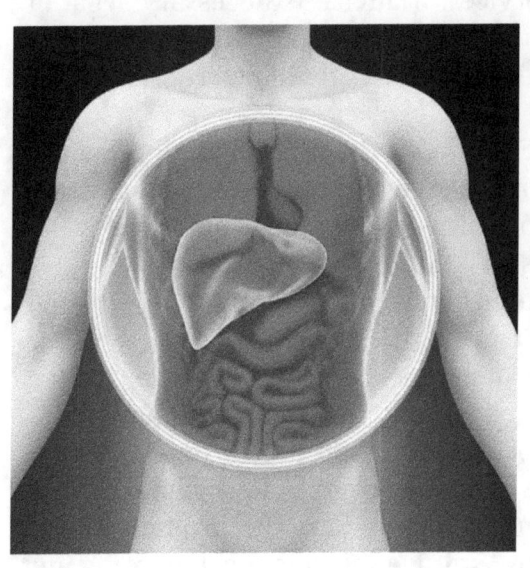

By
Fhilcar Faunillan

Fhilcar Faunillan

owners themselves, not affiliated with this document.

TABLE OF CONTENTS

INTRODUCTION

Good day, reader! First and foremost, I would like to say thank you for deciding to purchase my book entitled, *"Loving Your Liver: Your Complete Guide to Prevent, Cure, and Reverse Fatty Liver."* It just shows that you are concerned about your body, specifically your liver. Congratulations, you have just made the first step to becoming healthier!

In the busy world that we are living right now, people tend to forget about keeping their bodies healthy. They just wake up, grab whatever they can to munch, rush to work, socialize after office hours, go home to doze off, and just call it a day. This cycle keeps going on every day for the rest of the week, the month, and eventually, the whole year. What happens to the importance of having a balanced diet and exercise? A lot of people often do not keep that in mind. What people do not understand is that while they enjoy this kind of lifestyle, they are gradually harming their bodies. This is why most people suffer from different diseases. One of the most common and sometimes alarming diseases is fatty liver.

Fatty liver can be obtained through various reasons. If you think the only victims of this disease are those alcoholic individuals, then you are wrong. Even non-alcoholic drinkers are exposed to the risk of having fatty liver. The increase in number of people having deteriorating liver have already caused an alarm. This is one of the reasons why liver health care is becoming quite popular nowadays. Due to our busy lifestyle, we most likely abuse our bodies without even really thinking about it. In most cases, people who acquire fatty liver do not even realize they have it. Symptoms of fatty liver often do not appear at first. In many instances, these become noticeable after years or even decades. Have you ever wondered if perhaps you could get this disease?

To answer that question, consider answering this set of questions first:

Have you experienced unusual . . .

- tiredness?

- loss of weight or appetite?

- weakness?

- nausea?

- confusion, poor judgment, or trouble concentrating?

- pain in the abdomen, especially in the upper-right side, just below the ribs?

If you answer yes to all of the questions, then I guess we have some sort of a greasy situation going on inside your body. The questions being asked are some of the notable problems people experience when having fatty liver. But do not fret so much about it because you now have this book. You have definitely made the right decision to purchase this book. This book will teach you what you need to know about fatty liver. Read onto the following chapters to learn what you can do about having fatty liver.

Once again thank you for downloading this book and happy reading!

Chapter 1 - What is Fatty Liver?

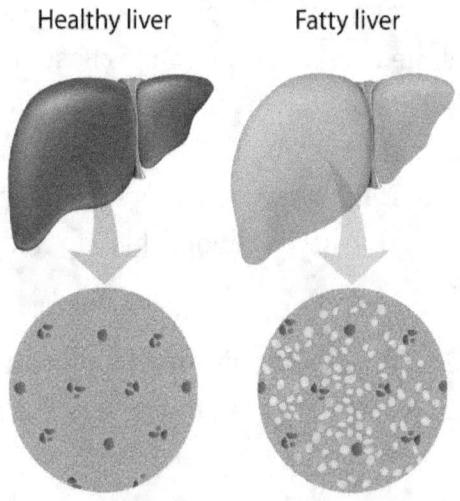

Healthy liver   Fatty liver

Before we talk about fatty liver, we must first understand the basic features and functions of our liver. The liver is considered one of the largest internal organs of the human body. It is located on the upper-right side of the abdomen. One of the major functions of the liver is removing toxins, like alcohol, and bacteria in our body.

Another of its major function is processing nutrients in the food we consume. The liver produces bile which helps in the digestion of food. Bile is stored in the gallbladder in between meals. When a person eats, it is secreted through the bile ducts - which connects the gallbladder and liver to the small intestines. The bile's job is to break down fats from the food we take into fatty acids. These are then taken into the body by the gastrointestinal (GI) tract, or mostly known as the digestive tract. The GI tract is made up of hollow organs namely: the mouth, esophagus, stomach, small intestine, large intestine (including the rectum), and the anus. While those are the "empty" parts of the digestive system, the liver, pancreas, and gallbladder are considered as the solid organs. The liver first filters blood from the digestive system before it can go freely to anywhere else in our body. It acts like a factory which makes vital substances such as albumin, which is a protein in our blood plasma, and other factors that help our body's ability of coagulation, or blood clotting. Moreover, the liver collects and stores essential substances, such as sugar and vitamins, which will be used by the body later.

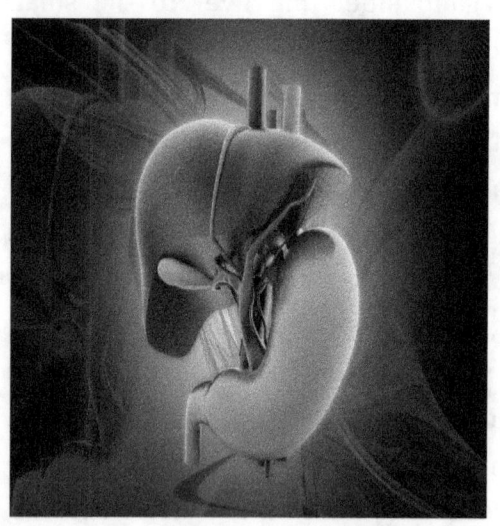

To sum it all up, the liver's job is:

- converting food into energy and producing chemicals that are needed by your brain and spinal cord

- controlling blood clot and cholesterol production and excretion, and regulating stored fat

- producing bile – which is a substance that helps in digesting food and absorbing essential nutrients

- cleansing your system by absorbing and secreting toxins such as drugs, alcohol, and other environmental poison in the body

- assisting in fighting off infections by generating immune factors and removing bacteria from the blood

- storing essential vitamins, minerals, and energy which are released into the blood as soon as these are needed

Now that we already have an idea what our liver does, we can now talk about the disease it can accumulate, which in this case is fatty liver.

Fatty liver disease, which is also known as steatosis, is a condition in which there is an abnormal increase in the amounts of fat that are accumulated by the cells of the liver. According to statistics, it affects one in every ten people and is mostly complained about in Western countries. Although it is important that the liver contains an amount of fat, it becomes unhealthy when the fat content is more than ten percent (10%) of the weight of the liver. This much amount of fat clearly makes you positive for having a fatty liver. If not taken care of immediately, you may experience more serious complications.

To understand more clearly about fatty liver disease (FLD), you must know that FLD has three (3) types. These are named: (1) alcoholic fatty liver, (2) non-alcoholic fatty liver, and (3) acute fatty liver of pregnancy. No need to worry, we will talk about each type so that we could have a full understanding of the different types of liver disease.

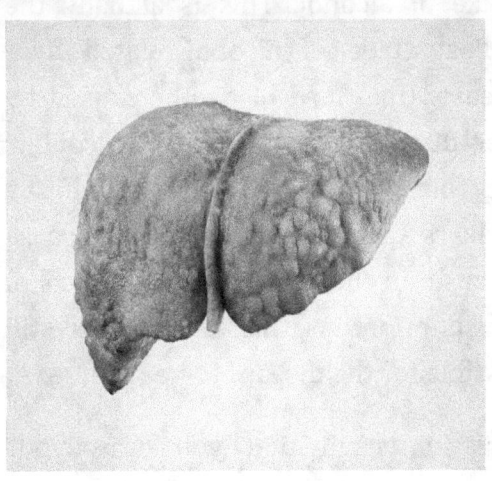

Alcoholic Fatty Liver Disease

As the name suggests, alcoholic fatty liver disease (AFLD) is a type of FLD which is apparently caused by the intake of alcohol. This is actually the earliest stage of alcohol-related liver disease. One-third of deaths caused by liver disease is accounted to alcoholic fatty liver disease. A lot of heavy drinkers acquire fatty liver disease because of having too much alcohol consumption. At this point, it is still possible for the disease to be reversed.

It is important that you draw your attention to your liver once you get the early signs of having an alcoholic fatty liver disease, especially when you know that you are inclined to drinking alcohol. If you are lucky enough to be diagnosed during its early stage, then you may still have the chance to cure and reverse the disease. Otherwise, you are in great risk of having liver failure and ultimately, death since this disease can rapidly jump from one bearable stage to a less tolerable one. To know more of this disease, read on to the next chapters.

Non-Alcoholic Fatty Liver Disease

While most people relate liver damage to abuse of alcohol or hepatitis, there is still an obscure and rampant liver condition that constitutes to an even greater threat to the health of the public. About one-third of the U.S. population suffers from a common but unnoticeable liver disease known as non-alcoholic fatty liver disease or NAFLD, in which alcohol has not been included as a cause. Most victims of this disease do not know that they have it. This disease may go unobserved for years and only appears when it has gone worse. NAFLD usually occurs to people who are overweight or obese. Diagnosis of NAFLD includes blood test. If results of the examination reveal that there is fat present in the liver, but without inflammation, then the patient most likely has a non-alcoholic fatty liver disease.

The importance of having the basic knowledge of non-alcoholic fatty liver disease is because of the fact that it has becoming a common disease at the present time. Moreover, its occurrence is gradually increasing. As a matter of fact, NAFLD has been linked with other serious and very common diseases that are not even liver-related, in which cardiovascular disease is considered to be the most important among others. This leads to heart disease and strokes, which are indeed fatal.

Acute Fatty Liver Of Pregnancy

The occurrence of the disease called acute fatty liver of pregnancy or what is known as AFLP, is usually a rare complication when one gets pregnant. However, this can be life-threatening. Not only to the mother, but also to the fetus inside the mother's womb. This usually occurs during the third trimester or in the early postpartum period. AFLP is described by micro vesicular fatty infiltration of hepatocytes – the major type of cells that makes up liver mass – but without inflammation or necrosis, or the death of a body tissue. It was first regarded as an acute yellow waste of the liver.

AFLP is prevalent in roughly one out of 10,000 to 15,000 pregnancies. Women who are pregnant are advised to be examined for the uncertain possibility of acquiring this fatal condition. This could lead to failures of the liver or kidney, which could either happen to the mother or the baby. In addition, AFLP might also be the source of infection or bleeding.

Now that we have identified and briefly explained the types of fatty liver disease, let us now proceed to finding out the causes, symptoms, and diagnosis of the disease which will be discussed in the following chapter.

Chapter 2 - Symptoms, Causes and Diagnosis

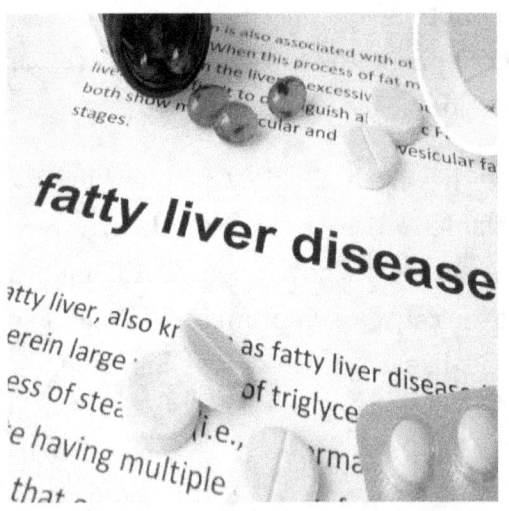

Do you want to know whether or not you are a victim of fatty liver disease? Then you must continue to read onto this chapter. This chapter talks about the things you need to know about the possible signs and causes of the different types of fatty liver disease. But before we proceed to discussing about the symptoms and causes of fatty liver, let us first talk about some common liver myths and facts.

Myth #1: *Alcoholics are the only victims of liver disease.*

Fact #1: Alcohol drinkers are not the specific victims of liver disease. There are actually more than a hundred causes of liver disease. The most common cause of abnormal liver tests conducted in the U.S. is accounted to non-alcoholic fatty liver disease, which does not have any connection with long or excessive consumption of alcohol. People who are mostly in risk of NAFLD are those who are obese, have diabetes, and have abnormally high levels of cholesterol and triglycerides (fats) present in their blood.

Myth #2: *The liver can only be damaged by an excessive amount of alcohol intake.*

Fact #2: Any amount of alcohol consumed can yield damage to the liver since alcohol is a harmful substance. What the recommendation of The National Institute of Alcohol Abuse and Alcoholism means by moderate drinking is that women should not have more than one drink per day, while no more than 2 drinks per day for men. Note that one drink is equivalent to either one 12-ounce bottle of 5% alcohol wine cooler or beer, one 5-ounce glass of 12% alcohol wine, or 1.5 ounces of 80-proof distilled spirits.

Myth #3: *It is useless to stop drinking alcohol when one has advanced liver disease.*

Fact #3: Discontinuing the intake of alcohol, even when one had advanced liver disease, is still helpful for the victim. According to frequent studies, those people who suffer advanced liver disease (cirrhosis) and still continuously consumes alcohol have only 33% chance of surviving in a span of 5 years compared to those who stopped, which accounted for 65%.

Myth #4: *Fat people are the only ones affected of fatty liver.*

Fact #4: People who are thin or those who have an average build can also have the chance of getting fatty liver. Even though people have no health problems in the nature of diabetes or obesity, they can still develop fatty liver. Fatty liver is acquired by having an unhealthy lifestyle, which would cause the accumulation of fat deposit build-up in the cells of the liver. Thus, it does not necessarily relate to one's current built.

I bet you got corrected with some of the myths that you were told to believe before. Now that we got those things cleared, let us now proceed to the things we should know regarding fatty liver.

Symptoms

You ought to know that fatty liver disease hardly ever shows symptoms until it has become far advanced. Patients with fatty liver are usually either asymptomatic – meaning showing no symptoms – or has symptoms but are not really specific and do not suggest acute liver disease. Typically, fatty liver is found or suspected:

• during routine liver blood testing, results are found to be abnormal

• when hepatitis are ruled out

• when performing ultrasonography of the abdomen, in cases of diagnosis of gallstones, fat is seen

- during physical examination of a patient, the liver is enlarged infrequently

Early symptoms of both *alcoholic* and *nonalcoholic fatty liver disease* may include the following:

- abdominal pains

- diarrhea

- elevated liver enzymes

- fatigue

- nausea

- vomiting

- weakness

When early symptoms are not paid attention to, the previously mentioned types of fatty liver diseases may become more serious. Symptoms may be found in the list below:

- anorexia

- bleeding in the gut

- dark colored patches on your neck and under your arms

- easy bruising

- fatigue

- increased sensitivity to alcohol and drugs (both medical and recreational since the liver can no longer process them)

- itching

- jaundice (having yellow skin)

- liver cancer

- loss of appetite

- swelling of the legs, ankles, or abdomen

- vomiting blood

- weakness

- weight loss

As what we have discussed in the earlier chapter, *acute fatty liver of pregnancy* usually starts to occur towards the end of the third trimester period, or the last three months, of pregnancy. Among AFLP's most common symptoms include the following:

- confusion

- headache

- jaundice (yellow coloring of the skin, eyes, and mucous membranes)

- nausea

- malaise or general discomfort

- pains in the abdomen, especially in the upper right side

- tiredness

- vomiting

As what you can see, the symptoms of AFLP may easily look like any other medical condition. However, considering that one is pregnant when having this disease, it is always best to consult a doctor for a diagnosis.

Causes

The most common cause of fatty liver is alcoholism or drinking too much alcohol. This is especially true for *alcoholic fatty liver disease*, obviously. Most, if not all, heavy drinkers of alcohol are victims of fatty liver disease. If you are a man, drinking more than eight units a day (four pints of 4% beer) for two to three weeks would most likely result to the development of fatty liver. If you are a woman, drinking over 5 units a day (a couple of 175 ml glasses of wine) would lead likewise. Alcohol has an impact on the way liver handles fat that enters in your body, which would make your liver cells get fully stuffed of it. When this happens, you may experience an ambiguous feeling of discomfort in your abdominal area because by then, your liver is swollen. This also leads to feeling nauseous and losing your appetite. Another possible cause of AFLD is genetics. The genes that are passed down from your parents may have a role in having this disease. They can impact the chance of you being an alcoholic. Furthermore, they can also affect the way your body breaks down the alcohol you consume.

There is a rapid increase of the incidence of *nonalcoholic fatty liver disease* in the U.S. which according to statistics, constitute 10-20% of the

American population. For non-alcoholics, NAFLD comes out as a common cause of function impairment of the liver. It is also mostly associated with being overweight or obese. Due to the increased amounts of fat which are removed from the blood and/or produced by the liver cells, not enough amounts are disposed of or exported by these cells, which results to fat accumulation in the liver. This highly increases the risk of having diabetes or high cholesterol, in which both can cause fatty liver disease as well. This disease is more likely to happen to middle-aged people who are obese. However, because of the alarming increase in childhood obesity, children may also be victims of this disease. To know whether or not you are obese, calculate your Body Mass Index (BMI) using this formula:

BMI = weight in kilograms divided by (height in meters)^2

For example, if you are 1.80 meters tall and weigh 105 kilograms, BMI = 105 / $(1.80)^2$ = 32.40. To know what that figure signifies, we have to take note that having a BMI of less than 18.5 is classified as underweight; 18.5 to 24.9 is the normal weight; 25 to 29.9 is classified as overweight; obese I is 30 to 34.9; followed by 35 to 39 as obese II; and obese III is BMI of 40 or higher.

Referring to the table, our example would mean that you are on the first level of obesity. This would further connote that you are at risk of having NAFLD. Other causes of NAFLD may include starvation and protein malnutrition, the long term usage of total parenteral nutrition (a feeding procedure involving direct nutrient infusion into the blood stream), intestinal bypass surgery for obesity, rapid weight loss, and side effects of medications along the lines of aspirin, steroids, tamoxifen, and tetracycline.

Similar to AFLD, NAFLD may also be caused by genetic factors.

Up to this point in time, no one still fully understands the exact cause of fatty liver which occurs during pregnancy. However, according to research, hormones may contribute to such disease which leads to an abnormality in the metabolism of fetal fatty acids. In addition, recent studies say that *acute fatty liver of pregnancy* may be caused by a mitochondrial dysfunction during oxidation of fatty acids in the liver. The process of mitochondrial oxidation normally consists a series of transport steps with four enzymatic reactions. Victims of AFLP lack the third enzyme, which helps in breaking down a long chain of fatty acids.

Diagnosis

During a blood test or a routine check-up, your doctor might notice something unusual or see that your liver is slightly enlarged than usual. Although mild, these could be some signs of having a fatty liver. To make sure that you do not have more probable liver diseases, your doctor might ask you to undergo more tests.

One way to diagnose fatty liver is through a physical examination. In cases where the liver has become inflamed, your doctor can detect it by examining your abdomen. It can reveal that you may have historically experienced fatigue or loss of appetite. It may also reveal a history of your involvement in alcohol, medication, and supplement use. Another way of diagnosing fatty liver is through blood tests. A high number of liver enzymes found in blood tests could mean that you have fatty liver. However, this does not necessarily confirm that you have such. This still needs further analysis to find out the cause of inflammation. Ultrasound may also be a means to diagnose fatty liver. This generates sound waves that are emitted into the body which then causes echoes returning and are recorded in order to "visualize" the structures beneath the skin. The reflected echoes from a variety of tissues which are measured creates a shadow picture. The fat inside your liver will appear as a white area on the recorded image. Similar imaging studies may be done as well. These are through computed tomography (CT) scan and magnetic resonance imaging (MRI) scan. CT scan produces combined X-ray images using computer technology to show three-dimensional images of the internal organs and structures of the body. It is used to define normal and abnormal structures in the body. Considered an important technique in radiology, an MRI scan makes the use of magnetism, radio waves, and a computer to generate images of body structures. The imaging results of MRI are more detailed and have a higher resolution than that of a CT scan. The last known procedure for diagnosing fatty liver is liver biopsy. After the doctor numbs your abdominal area with local anesthetic to lessen the pain, a needle is inserted through your skin and extracts a sample tissue from your liver for examination. The piece of tissue is then examined under a microscope. This is the only certain way of knowing whether or not you have fatty liver. Signs of fat, inflammation, and damaged liver cells are checked if present or not. The biopsy will also help in determining the exact cause of your disease.

Chapter 3 - How Can You Prevent Fatty Liver?

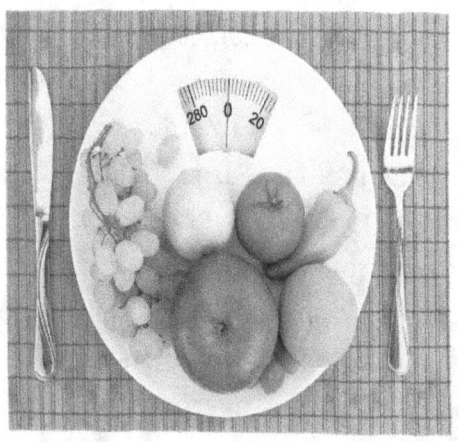

The only way to prevent yourself from acquiring fatty liver is to take good care of your liver. You only have a single liver in your body which plays an important role in your digestive system. Here are some ways to help keep your liver healthy:

1. Avoid drinking a lot of alcohol. Drinking excessive amounts of alcohol damages the cells of your liver and will lead to its swelling or scarring that will become cirrhosis in the long run. Cirrhosis is a slowly developing livedisease by which it replaces your healthy liver tissues with scar tissues. This will, in due course, prevents your liver from functioning as it should be. This will lead to liver failure and is fatal.

2. Eat a balanced, healthy diet. Limit your intake of food with high carbohydrates such as bread, rice, potatoes, corn, and grits. Before you start drinking, consider eating a healthy meal. Between drinks, eat low-fat, low-salt snacks to help your liver slow down the absorption of alcohol. Good nutrition brings help in supporting your liver to function well and plays a crucial role when it comes to your health.

3. Have a regular exercise. Consider exercise as a leisure rather than a burdensome activity. You can enjoy going for a walk in your neighborhood, swimming, gardening, or even as simple as stretching. It is important that you maintain a healthy weight.

4. **Cut down sugar and fats.** If you are a lover of sweet and fatty foods, you may consider slowly trimming it down. Minimize sugar consumption by limiting your intake than the usual. If you eat candies after every meal, you may perhaps only eat it once a day. If you are a candidate of diabetes, better only eat sweets once a week. Reduce your consumption of fried food as well, especially if you are a possible victim of high cholesterol.

5. **Be cautious of certain medicines.** Some drugs for cholesterol and the painkiller acetaminophen (Tylenol) may possibly hurt your liver if you take in too much doses. You may be taking more amounts of acetaminophen than you even realize. This is mostly found in a lot of drugs like cold medicine and prescribed painkillers. In some cases, medicines can hurt your liver when you drink alcohol while taking them. Some medicines are also harmful when they are combined with other drugs. To assure safety, consult your doctor or pharmacist on the ways of taking your medicines.

6. Drink coffee. Some studies have shown that drinking coffee has beneficial effects. The caffeine content in coffee, when consumed, lowers the occurrence of abnormal liver enzymes. This is associated with liver protection as well.

In order to keep your liver healthy, it is important that you follow a healthy lifestyle. Moreover, before you take medicines, be sure to have a consultation with a physician or pharmacist to make sure that you are in safe hands. The liver may be a very forgiving organ, but it also has limits.

Thus, you must be very careful not to abuse your liver. Have regular visits to a doctor who specializes in liver care to prevent yourself from getting fatty liver and even other worse conditions.

Chapter 4 - How Can You Cure Fatty Liver?

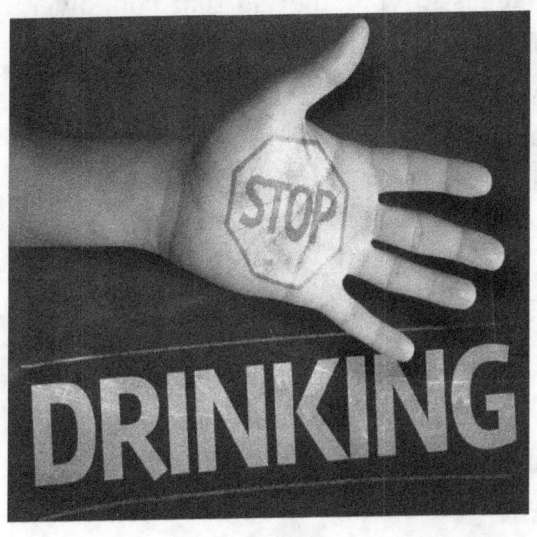

Failure to prevent fatty liver disease will lead you to experiencing the symptoms of the said disease, which clearly signals you to promptly visit a doctor for a check-up. After having been diagnosed of fatty liver, you may still save yourself from getting it worse.

One way of treating *alcoholic fatty liver disease* is requiring yourself to have a healthy diet, which includes avoiding alcohol. Once you get yourself checked up, your doctor may tell you to have changes in your diet so that your liver may recover from the damages caused by the alcohol you consumed. In most cases, in order to cure this disease, it may be necessary for you to participate in an alcohol recovery program. Furthermore, to deal with the complications caused by the damages in your liver, there may be a need for medications. For those victims with advanced AFLD who fail to improve with abstaining from alcohol and medical management, they may benefit from a liver transplant, which is their last resort. If you regularly drink more than the limits which are recommended, you might want to consider trying these simple tips to help cut down your alcohol intake:

1. **Make a drinking plan.** Before you begin drinking, set a certain limit on

how much you are going to drink for that day.

2. Set a drinking budget. On the occasion that you go out for drinking, only bring a fixed amount of money with you which you will use in spending for alcohol.

3. Let your loved ones know. When you let your family and friends know that you are cutting down on alcohol and that you will explain to them how much important it is to you, they will really be of good help in supporting you.

4. Take it one day at a time. Slowly cut down alcohol a little each day. That way, you will feel that you have achieved something every day.

5. Make servings into a smaller one. In the event that you want to revel in drinking, you can go for smaller sizes or amounts. Instead of having pints of beer, why don't you choose the bottled kind; or instead of a large glass of wine, go for a small one.

6. Choose a drink with lower strength. In place of strong beer or wines, cut down the alcohol by swapping them for ones with a lower strength, or lower percentage of alcohol by volume (ABV). Look for this information printed on the bottle's label.

7. Stay hydrated. Before you start drinking alcohol, drink a pint of water first. Never use alcohol as an alternative for water to quench your thirst. If you are not a fan of water, you can have a soft drink instead.

8. Take a break. Make sure to set an odd day in a week where you do not have to consume an alcoholic drink.

Patients with fatty liver who are obese are recommended to accomplish a steady and continuous weight loss. This can be achieved by taking in proper nutrition and having regular exercise. On the other hand, patients who have diabetes and contain high lipids in their blood have to increase their control of sugar and make sure that their lipid levels get lower. To lower the levels of blood sugar in people who have diabetes, it is highly advised that they go for a low fat, low calorie diet. This should be accompanied by insulin or other medications to help cure the fatty liver disease more quickly.

For those patients who have *nonalcoholic fatty liver disease* but are not overweight and do not have diabetes, oftentimes, a low fat diet is advised. Moreover, it is also suggested that they should refrain from drinking alcohol as it can be a major cause and a great contribution to having a fatty liver disease. People who have acquired fatty liver disease should see to it that they set an appointment to their primary healthcare providers on a regular basis.

To help cure fatty liver disease as soon as possible, it is very much essential that you should commit to change, and that means having your current lifestyle changed. Modern life makes it easier for us to eat and drink more than we actually realize but we only do a little physical activity despite consuming too much. This would more often than not result to having weight gain. Losing weight when you are overweight will definitely bring you a series of important health benefits. Do you want to know what the key to success is? It is by making realistic changes to your diet and the level of physical activity that you should consider to be part of your everyday routine. According to findings, it is evident that the best way to lose weight is to create changes in your diet and physical activity that would be good for a long term. With that, it would result to a steady rate in losing weight. Have an objective to lose around 0.5 to 1 kilograms of weight a week, which is about 1 to 2 pounds, until you could reach a healthy BMI of 18.5 to 24.9.

You need to alter your existing habits to be able to successfully lose weight. This would mean eating less – even when you are eating a healthy, balanced diet – and being more on the go. Those trending diets and exercises which are considered extreme are most unlikely to work for a long time. Although those would result to a rapid weight loss, those kinds of changes in your lifestyle can not be maintained in the long run. Once you decide to stop on those extreme programs, you are most likely to go back to your old habits and regain weight. Decide on changes on your diet and physical activity that you know you can include as part of your daily routine instead. Make sure to stick to it for life.

Are you ready to get started? Try doing some healthy things today. To know whether or not you need to lose weight, check your BMI using the table in chapter 2. If you are classified as overweight, consider the following tips:

1. Swap the next snack that you plan to eat for something that is healthier. Choose to have a piece of fruit, a fruit bun, or perhaps a slice of malt loaf with a low-fat spread. If you decide to keep doing this every day, then congratulations! You have just adopted your first habit in losing weight.

2. Now try to trade your drinks that contain high calories for drinks that have lower contents of fat and sugar. Exchange that carbonated drink full of sugar for a sparkling water with a slice of lemon. Also keep in mind that alcoholic drinks contain calories as well. So deciding to cut down your

consumption could give you the benefit to control your weight.

3. The next thing to do is to look for a way to fit just one extra walk into your day. It has been proven that brisk walking is an effective way to burn down calories, and you can usually have time to include this in your daily routine. You might want to consider taking a walk to some shops during your lunch break, or getting off one stop earlier from the bus on your way home and just walk the rest of the way. Commit to this tip and you have adopted your second long-term habit in losing weight. If at all possible, try aiming to walk ten thousand (10,000) steps a day. It is not actually that many as it sounds. Learn to love walking more for your health.

4. Lastly, try to think ahead regarding what you will eat for breakfast tomorrow morning. Would it be

possible to make it healthier using the foods that are available in your home?

Now that we are finished with what healthy things you ought to do today, let us try to aim some things to do for a weekly basis. For this week, consider doing the following:

1. Plan to go to a healthy shop weekly. The key to a healthy weight is to have healthy, balanced meals. The start of eating a balanced diet is to have the right foods available at your home. When you go to the supermarket to buy groceries, look out for fresh foods and choose healthier options.

2. Everyone likes an occasional treat, like pizza for instance, or any food to go. What you can do is to switch your treat for a homemade substitute which you can make healthier. When you prepare food, you can make versions which have lower calories than those take-out foods you buy from diners or eateries. If you

do decide to order food, choose the healthier offers.

3. The next thing you should do for this week is to commit to one more method of increasing the level of your physical activity. The right amount of exercise for you is dependent on how old you are. For adults aging between 19 and 64 years old, it is highly recommended that they get moderate-intensity aerobic physical activity even for at least 150 minutes. Activities such as brisk walking and cycling per week would be some of what you can do. In order to lose weight, you may need to do more exercises.

4. The last thing to do is for you to pinpoint this week's danger zones. There are instances wherein you find yourself eating plenty of foods that are rich in fat and sugar. It may be because you are eating out or simply due to the fact that you are just so tied or stressed

out. What you can do is to plan ahead so that you can limit those kinds of food. Nevertheless, do not be too hard on yourself. An indulgence of food from time to time is fine, as long as you know how to burn it out.

Include exercise as a part of your routine. Each week, try doing at least 150 minutes of moderate exercise, in sessions of 10 minutes or more. As an alternative, you may opt for a "vigorous-intensity" aerobic activity for 75 minutes, such as running or playing a game of tennis every week. You can also do muscle-strengthening activities on major muscle groups such as the abdomen, arms, back, chest, hips, legs, and shoulders on two days or more each week.

If you have been diagnosed with high cholesterol, your doctor will most likely advise you to change your diet and increase your levels of exercise. Making changes to your diet, deciding to stop from smoking, and exercising more will help in preventing the development of high cholesterol. Your level of low-density lipoprotein (LDL) or the bad cholesterol can be reduced when you choose to eat a healthy diet that is low in saturated fats. The following are foods rich in saturated fat which you must cut down or avoid:

• Fatty parts of meat and meat products like sausages and pies

• Butter or lard

• Cream, sour cream, and ice cream

• Cheese, especially hard cheese

• Cakes

• Biscuits and cookies

• Chocolate

• Coconut (oil and cream) and palm oil

As suggested by experts, the average man should only have at most 30 grams of saturated fat per day, while the average woman should have less than 20 grams a day. To make sure that you know how much content of saturated fat is in the food you eat, check out the food labels before you take a bite or sip.

Since fatty liver disease is associated with cardiovascular disease, you must keep in mind that it is also important to control your habits which can bring risk in having the latter disease. One fatal habit is smoking. If you smoke, you should know that it is significant to give up. Stopping yourself from smoking will help in reducing your chance of getting a heart attack and stroke. Many people who engage in smoking do not realize that their general practitioners (GP) can actually help them to quit smoking. They can enroll you in a "stop smoking" clinic, prescribe you some nicotine replacement therapy such as patches and gums, or even give you medication such as Champix. Since nicotine is addictive, controlling yourself from not smoking may not be enough. You might want to consider using nicotine replacement therapy (NRT) to have a better chance of quitting successfully. You can get it by a prescription from your GP. Otherwise, you may also purchase nicotine patches or gum over the counter in a pharmacy.

If you have been diagnosed with diabetes, there are three major areas that you need to look closely at: 1) diet, 2) weight, and 3) level of physical activity. By choosing to eat healthy, losing weight (if you are overweight according to your BMI), and including exercise as a regular part of your lifestyle, you may be able to keep a safe and healthy blood glucose level without needing to undergo other types of treatment.

According to medical practitioners, at the present time, there are no specific medicines to cure NAFLD. Nevertheless, certain medicines which are used to treat high cholesterol and diabetes are found to have a beneficial effect on the liver. Your physician may prescribe a specific medicine that will help you to reduce the incidence of having NAFLD which could cause cirrhosis or liver cancer. If you are diagnosed with high cholesterol and/or type 2 diabetes, it may be necessary to get medical treatment for these. Given that you have been eating a healthy diet and regularly exercising, in cases when after a few months your cholesterol and blood sugar levels have not decreased, you will typically be advised to take cholesterol- and blood sugar-lowering medications. There are various kinds of medication that work in many ways. Your doctor will advise you regarding the most suitable kind of treatment for you. Some of the common prescriptions are the following:

1. Statin. Statin's job is blocking the enzyme, a type of chemical that helps in making cholesterol, in your liver. This will result to a decrease in the level of your blood cholesterol. Like in most cases, your doctor will usually advise you to start with the drug named atorvastatin. Other statin drugs would include simvastatin and rosuvastatin. Since statins are usually needed to be taken for life, these are only prescribed to people who continuously have a high risk of heart disease. This is due to the fact that levels of cholesterol may start to rise again once you stop taking them.

2. Aspirin. Depending on the age and other factors, a low dose of aspirin every day may be prescribed by the doctor. You must know that children under 16 years old are not allowed to take aspirin. A low dose of aspirin can help in preventing blood clots and also stroke.

3. Niacin. Commonly known as Vitamin B3, Niacin is found in foods as a multivitamin supplement. Niacin reduces triglycerides and increases high-density lipoprotein (HDL) or the good cholesterol when taken in high doses, which is available by prescription. Niacin can be offered to people who have a high triglyceride level.

4. Metformin. This is usually the first drug prescribed to patients who have type 2 diabetes for treatment. It lowers the amount of glucose that is released into the bloodstream by the liver. Metformin also helps the cells of the body to be more responsive to insulin.

5. Pioglitazone (Actos) and rosiglitazone (Avandia). These drugs are prescribed to people who are suffering from diabetes because these increase sensitivity to insulin. Research has shown that signs of liver injury has been reduced, along with fat in the liver. Pioglitazone might also help to reduce scarring from liver inflammation.

6. Vitamin E. Studies have shown that it reduces liver fat and inflammation, and possibly fibrosis, which is the next stage of having fatty liver. However, its effectiveness and safety in the long run have not been studied well yet.

7. Omega-3 fatty acids. It has been believed by experts that the fats found in avocados and oily fish like mackerel, salmon, and tuna are beneficial for you. High doses of these omega-3 fatty acids can lower levels of triglyceride in some patients. On a side note though, too much consumption of omega-3 fatty acids can contribute to obesity. Only about two oily fish-based meals a week are considered to be beneficial for people who have a high triglyceride level. However, there has not been any proof about taking omega-3 supplements to have the same benefit.

8. Ezetimibe. This is a medication which blocks the process of absorbing cholesterol in your blood from the food you eat and the bile juices in your intestines. Although it is generally not effective as satins, it is less likely to cause any side effects.

When the previously mentioned treatments are not effective in curing fatty liver, other treatments are still available. These can be by means of:

1. Bariatric surgery. This is mostly done to obese or overweight people who have a hard time in losing weight. This is a surgery of the gastrointestinal tract which effectively results to weight loss. Since it has been believed that obesity is one important factor in the causality of having nonalcoholic fatty liver disease, it is quite expected that bariatric surgery has been considered as a possible cure for nonalcoholic fatty liver disease.

2. Liver transplant. Once the liver has progressed (gone worse) from being fatty to becoming cirrhotic and there will be further developed complications, the only options you can have are either to treat the complications as they appear or to replace the worn out liver with a transplanted one.

When it comes to *acute fatty liver of pregnancy*, it is a different story. This disease is more dangerous and fatal because not only the mother is affected, her child inside her gets affected as well. According to historical data, the death rate of mothers and fetuses were stated to be as high as 75% and 85%, correspondingly. But according to a later collection of data, it has shown that due to prompt diagnosis and treatment of AFLP, both maternal and perinatal mortality rates have significantly decreased. It has now become 18% and 23%, respectively. In spite of the data gathered regarding this condition, the exact pathogenesis – the manner of development of a disease – has not yet been identified. It is important to keep in mind that once you get a diagnosis of this disease, it is very much vital that your baby gets delivered as soon as possible. This is so far the best treatment at present. Both your and your baby's lives are at extremely high risk if AFLP will remain to be untreated. Complications such as liver and kidney failure, hemorrhage, and sever infection can be very fatal for the both of you. After the baby's delivery, you will possibly need intensive care for a couple of days. After a few weeks, however, your liver will oftentimes return to normal.

Curing fatty liver disease is one thing, reversing it is another. Now that we are done discussing about how the different types of fatty liver disease can be treated, let us now move on to the next chapter to talk about how to reverse such disease.

Chapter 5 - How Can You Reverse Fatty Liver?

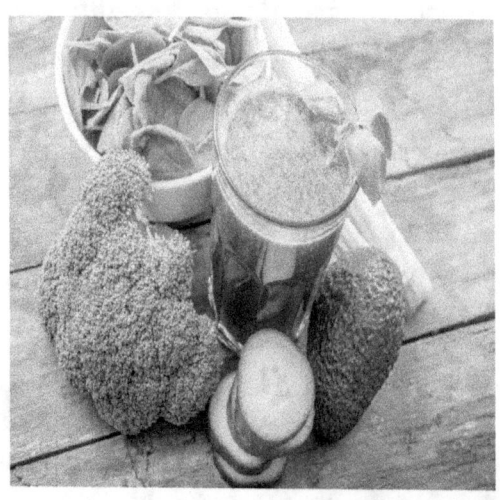

The damages that are caused by fatty liver disease can more often than not be ceased or reversed by making some simple lifestyle changes. In most cases, people who have fatty liver and have been diagnosed before conditions got worse, will not necessarily develop advanced liver disease. If the cause of fatty liver is associated with having high cholesterol, diabetes, or obesity, then treating those will reverse the whole fatty liver process. As what have been mentioned in the previous chapter, there is a cure for fatty liver. When you continue to do the guidelines to treat fatty liver, then lucky for you, the process could be reversed.

As a reiteration of the ways to cure fatty liver, here is a summary of what to do to achieve a successful reverse of fatty liver:

1. Eat less carbohydrates. An unhealthy diet leads to a cause of fatty liver disease. Most causes are your intake of sugar and foods made of white flour. It is necessary for you to completely avoid these. A large consumption of foods rich in carbohydrates can stimulate fatty liver since the liver converts excess carbohydrate into fat. Watch out for foods to be taken in limited amounts. These include pasta, rice, bread, potatoes, breakfast cereals, and any food made of flour. It has been proven that a low-carb diet burns more excess liver fat than a low-calorie diet.

2. Drink less alcohol. If the cause of your fatty liver is alcoholism, ending your habit of drinking will possibly allow your liver to completely heal itself. Abstinence of alcohol may reverse *alcoholic fatty liver disease.* To know how badly damaged your liver is from alcohol, a biopsy may be done.

3. Drink raw vegetable juices. You can get highly concentrated vitamins, minerals, and antioxidants from drinking raw juices. Your drink should contain 80-100% vegetables, and the remaining should be comprised of fruits.

4. Eat more vegetables, protein, and the right kinds of fat. The most powerful foods for healing the liver are raw vegetables and fruits. These raw foods are of great help in cleansing and repairing the liver filter, so that it would be able to trap and get rid of more fat and toxins from the bloodstream. Eat plenty of vegetable, both cooked and raw salads. While fruit is healthy for most people, it is best for those who have high blood sugar or resistance to insulin to limit themselves to 2 servings of fruit per day. Protein is essential to take in when having a fatty liver because it helps stabilize the level of blood sugar. It also helps in losing weight from the abdomen and minimizes hunger and cravings. It is advisable to have protein with each meal. Notable good sources of protein include nuts, legumes, seeds, eggs, poultry, seafood, meat, and dairy products such as cheese or milk. Other fruits and vegetables you may consider eating to help cleanse your liver are the following:

a. **Avocado.** This nutrient-dense fruit assists the body in producing glutathione, which is a compound necessary for the liver to rinse out harmful toxins.

b. Apple. Apples are high in pectin, which are chemical constituents that are needed by the body to cleanse and discharge toxins from the digestive tract. This makes it easier for the liver to hold on loads of toxins during the process of cleansing.

c. Beet and Carrot. Eating beets and carrots will help fuel and improve liver function since both of these are high in plant flavonoids and beta-carotene.

d. Broccoli and Cauliflower. These green vegetables increase the amount of glucosinolate in your system, which adds to the production of enzymes in your liver. These natural enzymes give the benefit of flushing out carcinogens and other toxins in your body which significantly lower your risk of having cancer.

e. Garlic. Even with just a little amount of this pungent white bulb, it can already activate liver enzymes that flush out toxins from your body. It is also rich in allicin and selenium, which are natural compounds that help cleanse the liver.

f. Grapefruit. This fruit increases the natural cleaning processes of the liver as it is high in vitamin C and antioxidants. Production of enzymes for liver detoxification will be boosted even with just a small glass of freshly-squeezed grapefruit juice.

g. Green, leafy vegetables. These are one of the most powerful foods that cleans the liver. Leafy greens may be eaten raw, cooked, or even juiced. These suck out the environmental toxins from your bloodstream since they contain extremely high amounts of chlorophylls. These are also considered as a protective mechanism for the liver due to its ability of neutralizing heavy metals and chemicals.

h. Green tea. This is full of catechins, a kind of plant antioxidant which is known to help in the functions of the liver. Green tea is also helpful in improving your overall diet.

i. Lemon and lime. These citrus fruits contain a high amount of vitamin C, which helps the body to synthesize toxic materials into substances that can be absorbed by water. Drinking lemon or lime juice in that is freshly squeezed in the morning aids in stimulating the liver.

a. Walnut. This helps in detoxifying ammonia from the liver. Also high in glutathione and omega-3 fatty acids, walnuts help in cleansing the liver.

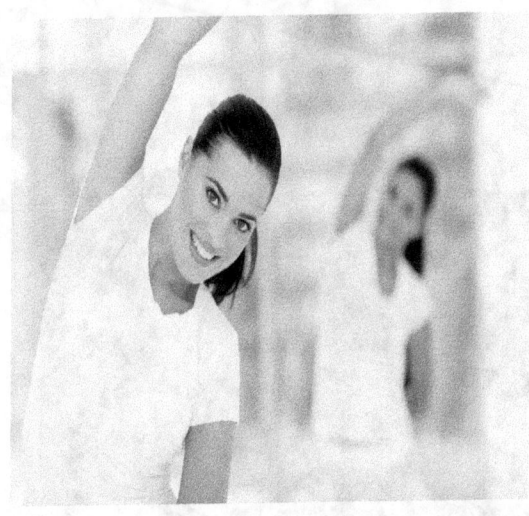

Exercise regularly. It is very much important to keep your body active so as to burn down fats, especially in your liver. Lose weight safely; meaning, you should lose no more than half to 1 kilogram (1 to 2 pounds) per week. To reverse fatty liver, aim to lose 20% of your current weight so as to reduce the inflammation and other damages done in your liver.

Chapter 6 - Why You Should Love Your Liver

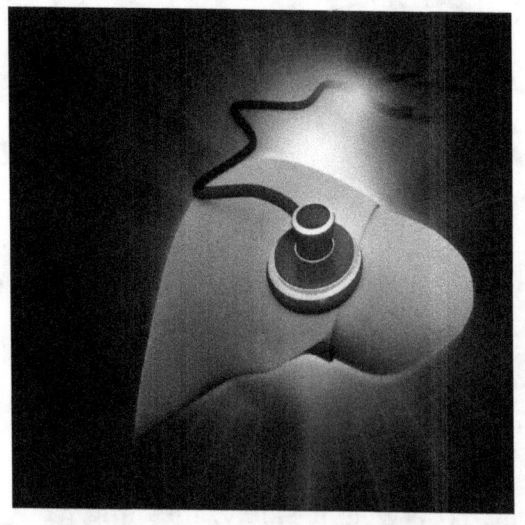

Aside from giving respect and accepting the body that you were born with, and of course taking care of it as best as you can, it is very much important that you consider the health of your vital organs as a top priority. You might ask, "Why bother?" Well, to answer that, is quite simple actually. Most of us, if not all, would like to live a happy and fulfilling life for as long as it is deemed possible. Although a lot may say having "quality" would be more preferred over "quantity", most of the time, it is during at the critical times of life that we would be able to realize that. When you are lying down there, waiting for when you can take in your last breath, you would most probably get to thinking whether or not you have lived enough to say goodbye.

Imagine someone who is dying due to the need of having a new liver. As much as they would hope that there would be a liver available to them so that their life would somehow be prolonged, it is not guaranteed that there is any. It is due to the brutal fact that for someone to be saved, someone else has to lose their life so their liver may be donated. Now that would not be a good scene. You do not want that to happen to you, do you?

Once a liver has been made available for a transplant, it is not that easy to proceed with surgery. There would still be tests to undergo. It is extremely important to match the new liver to the recipient according to its size, blood group, and if it is healthy enough with no further problems when being transplanted to the patient. After all, it is not always guaranteed that a matched liver is guaranteed. So once a new liver is available, this might be the only chance for the recipient to have a second life.

Indeed, the scenario I just presented was very straightforward. But try to imagine if there was not any suitable liver available, though, and your spouse, child, or parent was lying down on the hospital bed just waiting while their liver continues to deteriorate. You may be asked by the doctor if you or any other family member, or even a friend, would consider donating some part of your own liver. Given no other choice, you might as well volunteer to donate yourself in the hope to save your loved one's life. You might not realize that this is the only chance they got so you might as well take that one chance.

But consider a situation that might be tragic, but not at all impossible. After submitting yourself for some tests before you could donate, it was found out that your liver was not very healthy. They could still proceed with the operation though, but it would rather be more ideal if the liver would have been in a better condition so as to enable the recipient to have the best conceivable result. An even worse case scenario is being told that your liver had some disease of its own and thus it would be impossible for you to donate some part of it. How would you feel about that? I hope by giving you a clear picture of what might happen, you would be able to think back of what you could have done to keep your body a bit better. What I am really trying to say here is that not only you, yourself, could benefit from taking good care of your liver but also because someone else might just need a bit of it, and you could be the only possible donor.

The liver is not only an organ that helps in digesting our food as we are repeatedly taught in school, it also helps in detoxification where it cleanses our bodies from poisonous substances. Getting fatty liver, especially when it is not due to alcohol, is linked with other non-liver diseases that are very common yet serious. Perhaps the most alarming is cardiovascular disease that may lead to heart disease and strokes. Although fatty liver is not likely the cause of having the mentioned diseases, it is still but a manifestation of an underlying cause that most diseases share. Having fatty liver thus gives us a clue of the presence of these other fatal diseases which clearly need to be addressed as soon as possible.

You should love your liver simply so you could have a longer life to delight in. Keep in mind that you only have one liver and it would indeed be very unfortunate for you to lose it because your life depends on it. Having a healthy liver means having greater chances of doing the most of what you enjoy. Besides, it would be more costly to get sick rather than avoiding to get sick, which you can start off by choosing to have a healthy lifestyle. Remember, you are an important person. You might not realize it but a lot of people actually care about you. They value you so you must take good care of yourself so as to avoid any health complications. If you will not, then who else will?

CONCLUSION

Thank you again for downloading this book!

The consequences of not taking care of your liver would include obesity, a higher rate of having cardiovascular disease, continuing fatigue, headaches, problems with digestion, allergies, and a lot more conditions. Although our immune system protects our body from any harm, it is still the job of the liver to protect our immune system from overload.

A lot of people suffer from unnecessary weight and slow metabolism. As they age, they find out that they gain more weight bit by bit, and they just accept to have bulging stomachs and obstinate fat deposits. Although they have been dieting for years, it is still not enough for them to feel long-lasting relief. There must be something missing since this is obviously not right. Doctors say that the liver must be the missing key. It is, after all, the ultimate organ of metabolism. They have also pointed out that one must always consider the state of the liver when it comes to restoring good health.

Remember that the liver is the major organ that burns fat in the body. If you just follow the guidelines aforementioned, you will surely improve rapidly and begin to burn fat. On the contrary, if you choose to eat the wrong kinds of food, your liver would rend to build up more fats, which would result to storing more fat. On a bigger picture, it is not really about how much you eat, but it is rather what you eat that is far more important. By simply following the tips laid down for you in the earlier chapters, your liver will surely be relieved and get on with its job of controlling metabolism and burning down fat. The action of losing weight will then begin naturally and it would require less effort on your part.

Just to be sure, these are the things that you must remember:

• Fatty liver is caused by fats building up in the liver which brings damage in the organ and may lead to serious complications.

• Dangerous factors include obesity, having a high-fat diet, taking in excessive alcohol, and diabetes.

• People with fatty liver disease are highly recommended to change their current diets, do regular exercise, and shred off weight.

I must say, we have just come to an end of this book. Thank you for taking your time to read and learn about your liver and what disease it could seriously get. I hope this book is of great help to you as you choose to become a healthier person than you ever were. Once again,

I would like to say how grateful I am for choosing to purchase this book, and hats off to you as well for being able to finish reading the book and deciding to live a healthier life. Well done, my dear! Now, get up and get yourself working for a healthier liver. Choose to love your liver; your life depends on it.

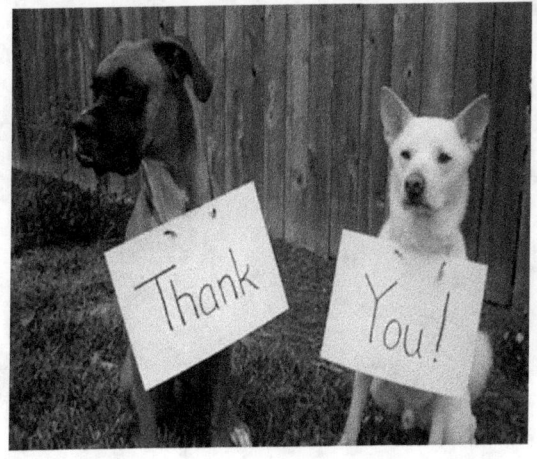

Finally, if you enjoyed this book, then I'd like to ask you for a favor, would you be kind enough to leave a review for this book on Amazon? It'd be greatly appreciated! Thank you and good luck!